contents

■ POLICIES AND PROCEDURES

Always follow your organisation's policies and procedures. It is your responsibility to make sure you keep up to date with any changes in these.

■ WHO TO CONTACT

Your local Primary Care Trust will employ an infection control team or nurse. You can find out their contact details via the PCT website or phone.

Where to go for further information:
- Department of Health website www.dh.gov.uk
- Medical Devices Agency
- National Institute for Health and Clinical Excellence (NICE) www.nice.org
  - NICE infection control guidelines
- National Patient Agency www.npsa.nhs.uk
- The RCN's guidance for nursing staff
  - Good practice in infection control
  - Methicillin-resistant *Staphylococcus aureus* (MRSA)

■ STANDARD UNIVERSAL PRECAUTIONS

Simple precautions that can be taken that minimise the risk of infection and so protects staff and patients. Universal precautions apply to everyone, everywhere. We all have a responsibility to minimise the risk of infection by making sure we take these precautions.

introduction

Standard universal precautions

- Clean hands – wash hands properly.
- Use protective equipment.
- Dispose of sharps and clinical waste safely.
- Manage blood and bodily fluids safely.
- Keep equipment uncontaminated.
- Maintain a clean clinical environment.
- Manage accidents and spills appropriately (following guidelines, policies and procedures).

Top tips for infection control

- Follow standard universal precautions:
  - effective hand washing;
  - use of protective clothing;
  - disposal of waste.
- Identify risk.
- Take appropriate action.
- Keep yourself and others safe.
- Follow local policies and procedures.
- Keep up to date with new developments.

How to wash your hands

■ ROYAL COLLEGE OF NURSING (RCN) GUIDE TO HAND WASHING

Hand washing technique

1 Palm to palm

2 Right palm over left dorsum and left palm over right dorsum

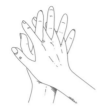

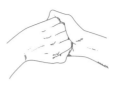

3 Palm to palm fingers interlaced

4 Backs of fingers to opposing palms with fingers interlocked

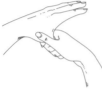

5 Rotational rubbing of right thumb clasped in left palm and vice versa

6 Rotational rubbing, backwards and forwards with clasped fingers of right hand in left palm and vice versa

Reference / Royal College of Nursing, Hand Washing Technique Chart, Publication 002 276. Reproduced by permission.

■ HAND WASHING BASICS

- Prepare by wetting the hands under running tepid water and apply liquid soap.
- Rub hands together for a minimum of 10–15 seconds making sure the hand wash solution comes into contact with all surfaces of the hand. Pay special attention to between the fingers and the base of the thumbs, not forgetting the wrists.
- Dry thoroughly with paper towels, dispose after single use.

■ WHY DO WE NEED TO WASH OUR HANDS?

- Hand washing is the single most important activity for reducing the spread of disease.
- Soap and water remove 99% of transient bacteria.
- Alcohol hand-rub kills 99.9% of transient bacteria.
- Where possible alcohol hand-rub should be used on clean hands as this gives the best protection.

■ REMEMBER TO DRY YOUR HANDS THOROUGHLY

- Dry palms and backs of hands.
- Work towel between fingers.
- Dry around and under nails.

This is important for the following reasons:

- Wet hands carry bacteria and they can become chapped and sore, the skin can be broken and cuts can become infectious and you can transfer this infection to others.
  - ○ Fingernails should be kept short and clean. Jewellery, especially rings with stones, wristwatches and bracelets should not be worn.
  - ○ Any cuts and abrasions should be covered.
  - ○ There are products available that can help protect your hands from becoming sore. These are barrier creams and protective film barriers.

■ WHEN TO WASH HANDS

- before and after starting work;
- before and after each patient contact;
- after going to the toilet;
- when going and coming back from breaks such as lunch;

- after handling dirty and/or infected linen;
- before handling food and drink.

References / Adapted from *NCFE Certificate in Infection Control*, York: Tribal Education and Royal College of Nursing (2004) *Good Practice in Infection Control: Guidance for Nursing Staff*, London: RCN, publication code 002 278.

■ HOW TO GET VISITORS AND STAFF TO COMPLY WITH HAND HYGIENE REQUIREMENTS

- staff member standing on duty near ward entrance at beginning and end of visiting time;
- audit;
- voice activated gel dispensers (that remind people who pass by to use the gel);
- patient and carer/visitor education about hand hygiene is essential.

Use of protective equipment

■ PERSONAL PROTECTION – PERSONAL PROTECTIVE EQUIPMENT (PPE)

All equipment should be handled as little as possible and changed between patients and procedures. It should be discarded immediately after use.

■ GLOVES

Wear gloves when there is a potential for soiling your hands with body fluids. Gloves must conform to European Community Standards and are for single use. Powdered and polythene gloves should not be used for healthcare procedures. An alternative to rubber latex gloves should be available for staff that are allergic to these.

Gloves should be worn:
- when handling blood, body fluids, secretions and excretions;
- for invasive procedures.

Gloves should be:
- disposed of in clinical waste.

Hands should be washed/gelled following removal of gloves

Putting on gloves

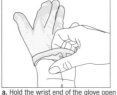

a. Hold the wrist end of the glove open and ease the fingers of the other hand inside

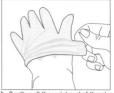

b. Gently pull the wrist end of the glove while easing the hand inside

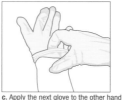

c. Apply the next glove to the other hand making sure to use the same procedure

Reference / Jeanes, A. (2005) Putting on gloves, *Nursing Times*, 101(29); Figures 1, 2, and 3. Reproduced with permission.

■ PLASTIC APRONS

Plastic aprons are for single use only.

Aprons should be worn:
- if there is a risk of being splashed, splattered or sprayed with bodily fluids:
  - ○ blood;
  - ○ secretions and excretions.

To remove aprons safely
When aprons are removed this should be done as follows:
- Break the plastic band behind the neck.
- Untie or break the plastic ties around the waist.
- Fold the apron inwards and roll from top to bottom (do not swing the apron about in mid air and do not allow the contaminated side to come in contact with your uniform).
- Dispose in clinical waste.

■ FULL FLUID REPELLENT GOWNS

Full fluid repellent gowns should be worn if there is a risk of extensive splashing for example as in child birth.

■ GOGGLES

Goggles should be worn to protect the eyes if there is a risk of bodily fluids splashing into the face or eyes.

■ MASKS

Masks should be worn where there is the risk of inhaling or coming into contact with body fluids. A mask may be needed if infection is spread by an airborne route for example multi drug resistant tuberculosis or serve acute respiratory syndrome (SARS). Masks should fit correctly and be handled as little as possible.

■ RESPIRATORY PROTECTIVE EQUIPMENT

Respiratory protective equipment should always be used when clinically indicated and the manufacturer's instructions should be followed when using and maintaining this.

■ UNIFORMS

Uniform is worn when working with the patients. Ideally it is worn only at the place of work, for example, health and social care workers wear their uniform in the hospital or care home in which they work, but not when they are journeying backwards and forwards to work; however this depends on whether there is a changing and locker room provided.

Uniforms should never be worn when the health and social care worker is not carrying out patient work, such as personal shopping or visiting a gym.

All too often even senior staff have been seen wearing their uniforms at inappropriate times. For those not provided with uniforms, washable clothes that are kept purely for work should be used and kept separate from other wear. For community workers ideally a coat should be supplied or a coat should be kept solely for work. The same applies for shoes.

If uniforms are washed at home, a 60 degree wash will kill most bacteria, if possible wash uniforms separately from other washing.

References / Adapted from Tribal Education (2006) *NCFE Certificate in Infection Control*, York: Tribal; Royal College of Nursing (2004) *Good Practice in Infection Control: Guidance for Nursing Staff*, London: RCN, publication code 002 278; National Institute for Health and Clinical Excellence (2003) *Guidelines for Infection Control*, London: NICE; and Reid-Searl, K., Dwyer, T,. Ryan, J., Moxham, L. and Richards, A. (2009) *Student Nurse Clinical Skills Survival Guide*, Harlow: Pearson.

Keeping yourself safe

- Wear gloves when there is a potential for soiling your hands. Always wash your hands once you remove your gloves.
- Wear goggles when there is a potential for being splashed or sprayed with bodily fluids.
- Wear a plastic apron where there is a risk of bodily fluids contacting your clothes.
- Wear a mask where there is a risk of inhaling body fluids.

■ WHAT TO DO IF YOU COME INTO CONTACT WITH BODILY FLUIDS

What to do if you come into contact with bodily fluids

Step 1
- Clean the area.
- If it is your skin, wash with soap and water.
- If it is a mucous membrane (such as your eye), wash with water or saline.
- If it is a sharps injury, wash with soap and water.

Step 2
- Report to your supervisor.
- Report to infection control team.
- Adhere to the organisation's policy and procedures.
- Seek medical advice (casualty if necessary).

Step 3
- Record incident on an accident form (or incident recording report).

Disposal of waste

■ MANAGING SHARPS
- Containers should meet British Standards 7320 or UN Standard 3291 and should be filled no more than to the line (approximately 2/3 full).
- Containers should be located in a safe position, and never on the floor (follow local policies).
- Sharps should be handled as little as possible.

- Do not pass sharps directly from hand to hand.
- Needles should not be re-sheathed.
- Do not break or bend needles.
- Do not disassemble needles/syringes/IV giving sets.

HINTS

Follow the organisation's policy and procedures when handling sharps. Sharps include needles, stitch cutters, scalpels, glass ampoules, any sharp instruments. The main hazard of a sharps injury is the risk of contracting hepatitis B, hepatitis C or human immunodeficiency virus (HIV). Blood-borne viruses are the second most common cause (after back injuries) of occupational injuries to health workers.

Reference / Royal College of Nursing (2004) *Good Practice in Infection Control: Guidance for Nursing Staff*, London: RCN, publication code 002 278.

Action to take following a needle stick injury

If contamination occurs take immediate action:

- Encourage bleeding by applying gentle pressure.
- Do not suck the wound.
- Wash affected area under running water.
- Dry area with a paper towel.
- Apply waterproof dressing.
- Report to infection control team.
- Seek medical advice.
- Report incident and record on accident or incident reporting form.
- Incident should be investigated and action plan devised to prevent reoccurrence taking place.

■ DISPOSAL OF CLINICAL WASTE

- Dispose of clinical waste in clinical waste bags.
- Bags should be filled to 2/3 full; tie bags securely and store in a designated clinical waste area.
- Place ripped or punctured bags inside another clinical waste bag.
- Store clinical waste bags in a secure area, until collected by the local authority.

■ LINEN

- Place uncontaminated linen in the clinical area in a white linen bag.
- Seal when no more than 2/3 full.

■ DEALING WITH INFECTED LINEN

Do not mix soiled linen with other laundry.

In the clinical area

- Deal with soiled and infected linen promptly.
- Place the soiled linen in a bag that is specifically identified as an infected linen bag, which are usually red in colour.
- Do not overfill the bags (fill to no more than 2/3 full) and secure with a tape.
- Bags are available that will dissolve on contact with hot water, these can then be placed directly into the washing machine and thus protect laundry staff from infection from handling the soiled linen.

In the client's home

- Flush any solid matter into the toilet.
- Wash soiled linen using pre-wash facility or cool rinse before main wash.
- Wash on hottest setting that the material will withstand, using detergent.

Decontamination of the environment and equipment

Most organisations will have formal education on how to decontaminate the environment and equipment for staff. The organisation will also produce policies and guidelines on this. Help with these can be obtained from the local infection control teams.

■ MEDICAL DEVICES

- Devices should be categorised according to the risk they pose for the patient.
- The risk is governed by the procedure rather than the instrument.

See Table below.

RISK	ITEM	RECOMMENDATION
LOW	• Not in contact with the patient • In contact with healthy skin	Clean with general purpose detergent or chemically disinfect if contaminated with body fluids

RISK	ITEM	RECOMMENDATION
MEDIUM	• In contact with mucous membranes or bodily fluids	Disinfection or single use
HIGH	• In contact with break in skin or mucous membrane • Or for equipment introduced into sterile body areas (e.g. surgical)	Sterilisation or single use

References / Adapted from Medical Devices Agency (1996) see Department of Health website, www.dh.gov.uk and Coventry PCT Infection Control Team.

Healthcare acquired infections

Healthcare acquired infections (HCIs) are infections that have resulted from care and treatment in a healthcare setting; these do not just occur in acute hospitals.

> **Healthcare acquired infections can occur in**
> - Hospitals
>   - Community
>   - Acute
>   - Specialist
> - Care homes
> - Assisted living
> - Hostels
> - Patient's own home.

Healthcare acquired infections include:
- Methicillin-resistant *Staphylococcus aureus* (MRSA)
- *Clostridium difficile* (C Diff)
- Septicaemia
- Gangrene
- Gastroenteritis
- Wound infections.

People who are at risk of acquiring healthcare associated infections include:
- The very old
- The very young
- Pregnant women
- Unborn children
- People with multiple health problems
- People with chronic diseases and long term conditions
- People who are immunosupressed
- People who misuse substances such as alcohol and drugs
- People living in poor social conditions.

■ METHICILLIN-RESISTANT *STAPHYLOCOCCUS AUREUS* (MRSA)

Methicillin-resistant *Staphylococcus aureus* is a big issue in healthcare acquired infections (in hospitals and in the community). MRSA causes pneumonia, septicaemia, wound infections, illness and death and should be prevented at all costs. Ways to do this are:
- Hand hygiene
- Use of protective equipment (aprons, gloves)
- Safe handling of equipment (patients' and staff equipment)
- Scrupulous cleanliness

- ○ Environment
- ○ Equipment
- Safe disposal of waste
  - ○ Sharps
  - ○ Laundry
  - ○ Used dressings
- Surveillance of patients, staff and visitors particularly during outbreaks
- Assessing and minimising the risks of developing MRSA
- Prompt treatment if it arises
  - ○ Seek assistance and advice from infection control team and microbiologist
  - ○ Use of appropriate antibiotics.

Managing MRSA hints
- Hand hygiene is very important.
- MRSA is spread mainly by hands.
- Scrupulous hand cleaning is needed to prevent MRSA from occurring and during outbreaks.
- Bacterial hand rubs should be also used (following washing and drying).

Taking extra care to manage MRSA
MRSA can be airborne so take care when
- making beds;
  - ○ do not shake bed clothes;
  - ○ keep bedclothes off the floor;
- careful containment and laundering of linen;
- thorough cleaning of beds, bed space, mattresses and equipment (such as moving and handling equipment);
- careful containment and disposal of waste.

Taking swabs for MRSA

Swabs may be taken from the following:

- Nose
- Throat
- Axillae
- Groin
- Perineum
- Wounds
- Urine.

Use an aseptic technique when taking the swabs

- if taking a swab from a wound, do this before cleaning or irrigating the wound;
- if there is no exudate the tip of the swab can be moistened with a transport medium or 0.9% sodium chloride.

Record patient details

- Name
- Date of birth
- Date and time swab taken
- Where swab was taken from (e.g. groin)
- Hospital number.

Reference / Nicol, M., Bavin, C., Bedford-Turner, S., Cronin, P. and Rawlings-Anderson, K. (2004) *Essential Nursing Skills*, Edinburgh: Mosby.

■ CLOSTRIDIUM DIFFICILE (C DIFF)

This bacterium is a normal component of the gut flora but can cause problems if it increases. First identified as a major cause of antibiotic associated diarrhoea causing mild to serious pseudomembranous colitis, it can cause serious illness and death.

> **Facts about C Diff**
> - Five per cent of healthy adults carry C Diff (in faeces) causing no ill effects.
> - Those at risk of serious illness from C Diff include:
>   - Older adults
>   - Young children
>   - Pregnant women
>   - Unborn children
>   - People with multiple health conditions
>   - People who have low immunities.
> - C Diff can cause death especially in the vulnerable groups (see above).

Aseptic technique

Aseptic technique is used to minimise the risk of infection. It is a technique using sterile equipment such as dressings and fluids.

■ PRINCIPLES OF ASEPTIC TECHNIQUE

- All equipment and dressings used must be sterile.
- Healthcare staff must wash their hands appropriately.
- All dressings and equipment should be handled with forceps or sterile gloves.
- All dressings and disposable equipment should placed in a closed container/bag and disposed of as clinical waste/sharps.

■ PREPARATION

The patient

- Explain what you intend to do.
- Gain consent, ensure person can understand you.
- Assess the wound.
- Check the person's comfort, such as, do they need to go to the toilet, are they in pain, etc.
- Make sure pain relief has had time to take effect.

The environment

- Clean dressing trolley or suitable surface.
- Collect dressing pack (intact and sterilised), cleaning solution, new dressings.
- Check that hand washing/decontamination facilities are available.
- Maintain privacy and dignity.
- Adjust bedclothes/person's clothes.
- Ensure area is clean and that any previous bed-making or cleaning of room etc. has taken place at least half an hour before proceeding.

Healthcare worker

- Consult care/treatment plan.
- Follow manufacturer's recommendations for dressings, solutions etc.
- Ensure uniform/clothes are clean.
- Ensure hair is clean and tied back.
- Wash and dry hands thoroughly.
- Wear a disposable apron.

The procedure

- Wash hands.
- Clean surface or trolley – follow local policies and procedures.
- Gather equipment, check dates, sterility, place on lower shelf of trolley.
- Wash and wipe scissors for cutting tape with an alcohol swab.
- Take trolley to the person.
- Adjust chair/bed to avoid unnecessary bending and stretching.
- Remove dressing pack from outer packaging and allow to drop on to top shelf of trolley.
- Attach clinical waste bag to trolley.
- Wash hands and apply alcohol gel.
- Carefully open dressing pack using just the finger tips.

References / Nicol, M., Bavin, C., Bedford-Turner, S., Cronin, P. and Rawlings-Anderson, K. (2004) *Essential Nursing Skills*, Edinburgh: Mosby and Bates (1971) *Paediatric Nursing*, Oxford: Blackwell.

■ COLLECTING SPECIMENS

Taking swabs

- Explain procedure to the patient and gain consent and co-operation (gain consent of appropriate adult).
- Ensure patient's comfort.
- Maintain patient's privacy and dignity at all times.
- Have appropriate equipment at hand:
  - Sterile swab
  - Specimen bag
  - Laboratory request form.
- Ensure the environment is suitable:
  - Private

- ○ Warm
- ○ Clean.
- Label swab.
- Wash and dry hands properly.
- Put on apron and gloves.
- Ask or assist patient to adopt position so swab can be taken.
- Open swab packaging at handle end.
- Remove swab (do not touch or contaminate the tip of the swab).
- Twist the swab so it comes into contact with the designated area.
- Avoid touching surrounding skin.
- Open transport tube and insert swab.
- Place in specimen bag.
- Make sure patient is comfortable.
- Despatch swab to laboratory and/or refrigerate as soon as possible.
- Dispose of waste.
- Remove gloves and apron – dispose.
- Wash hands.
- Document swab has been taken.

Reference / Adapted from Nicol, M., Bavin, C. and Bedford-Turner, S. (2004) *Essential Nursing Skills*, St. Louis, MO: Mosby.

Handling medication

- -

■ STORAGE OF MEDICINES

Medicines must always be stored at the manufacturer's recommended temperature. Some medicines need to be kept in a fridge; in a hospital or care home a separate lockable fridge should be used. This fridge should be maintained in accordance with the manufacturer's instructions (i.e. defrosted regularly), and be cleaned at regular intervals. If fridges are not maintained properly they will fail to function and medicines can lose their potency or become infected. All fridges used to store medicines should have a thermometer fitted, which should be checked regularly so that the correct temperature for storage is maintained.

Reference / Adapted from Tribal Education (2007) *NCFE Certificate in the Safe Handling of Medicines*, York: Tribal.

■ USE BY AND EXPIRY DATES

After opening, some medicines need to be discarded following a certain length of time. This time can vary as to the medication's manufacturer's instructions. Use by and expiry dates are provided because medicines can become contaminated with potentially harmful bacteria. These time limits must always be adhered to as should expiry dates. Re-using out of date medication or using medication for a longer period of time than what is recommended will result in harm to the person.

■ ADMINISTERING MEDICATION

Wash hands before commencing handling of medicines, when administering medication and following patient contact. Use the five rights and three checks:

Five rights
1. Right person
2. Right drug

3. Right dose
4. Right time
5. Right route.

Three checks
1. Check the label when getting the drug from storage.
2. Check the drug label with the prescription/drug order/ Medication Administration Record Sheet (MARS) sheet.
3. Re-check the drug prescription/order/MARS sheet after dispensing but prior to administration.

Reference / Reid-Searl, K., Dwyer, T., Ryan, J., Moxham, L. and Richards, A. (2009) *Student Nurse Clinical Skills Survival Guide*, Harlow: Pearson, p. 5.

General considerations to be taken into account when administering medication include
- Store all medicines as recommended by the manufacturer.
- Keep medication trolleys, cupboards, fridges, trays scrupulously clean.
- Gain patient's consent.
- Explain the purpose of the medication.
- Adhere to expiry and use by dates.
- Pay attention to special instructions such as avoiding alcohol, take after meals etc.
- Never leave medicines unattended.
- Nurses' role in self-administration of medicines is to support and educate the patient to give their own medicines especially with regards to minimising and controlling infection.
- Dispose of any packaging and other waste in appropriate way.
- Document your actions carefully and accurately.

Oral medication
- This is a clean procedure, wash and dry hands thoroughly.
- Adhere to expiry and use by dates.
- Clean bottles (and wipe following administration).
- Clean medicine spoons and pots.
- Dispense liquid medicine by pouring required amount in a clean medicine pot – a syringe may be used for accuracy.
- Dispense tablets/capsules into a medicine pot:
  - in a blister pack push tablet from the front of the pack, do not handle the tablet or capsule;
  - in a bottle shake required number of tablets/capsules into the lid of the bottle – do not handle these.
- Only soluble or dispersible medications should be dissolved in clean drinking water.
- Wash hands following direct patient contact (this should be done every time this occurs).

Medicine by subcutaneous (SC, sub cut) and intramuscular (IM) injection
- Packaging for equipment used should be intact and expiry date and sterility of packaging checked.
- Maintain patient's privacy and ensure their dignity.
- Wash hands before and after patient contact.
- Use aseptic technique to open the syringe and needle packaging and employ technique throughout the injection process.
- Do not touch top of opened ampoules or vials.
- Clean the rubber stopper of the ampoule with an alcohol-impregnated swab and allow to dry before inserting the needle.

- When mixing medicine, keep the needle inside the ampoule so that it remains sterile (otherwise change needle for a sterile one before injecting the patient).
- Needles must never be re-sheathed.
- With subcutaneous injections such as insulin, the skin is not cleaned with an alcohol swab as this can cause the skin to harden.
- Alcohol swabs will be used to clean the skin before intramuscular injections (allow the area to dry before commencing with the injection).
- Dispose of sharps appropriately.

Medicine by intravenous injection (IVI)
- Wash and dry hands.
- Prepare medicine for administration.
- Check cannula site for signs of infection, phlebitis or discomfort or pain. If site is bandaged, bandage should be removed to allow for inspection of site. If the infusion is running the medication can be administered via the injection port. The infusion should be stopped while medicine is administered and recommenced following this.
- Use aseptic technique when drawing up medications and when administering them – wash and dry hands.
- Disinfect the rubber membrane of the injection port (follow your organisation's policy for this).
- 0.9% sterile sodium chloride is used to flush (to confirm that the cannula is open) – if there is any resistance do not continue as this may cause a clot to dislodge.
- Slowly administer medicine (follow policy).
- Flush cannula between each medicine given.
- Flush cannula when all medicine has been given.

Administering eye drops and eye cream

- Arrange clean tissues or swabs to hand.
- Follow normal patient/medication checks.
- Wash and dry hands.
- Remove cap from drops or ointment container; do not touch the opened top.
- Hold tissue/swab beneath eye, gently pull down the lower lid.
- Hold dispenser about 2–3 cm from patient's eye.
- If drops and ointment are prescribed, apply drops first.
- Squeeze one drop into eye and ask patient to blink (some patients find it easier to look up) before administering more drops (administer as prescribed).
- Squeeze thin 'ribbon' of ointment on to lower inside of eyelid, from nose to ear.
- Do not let the container for drops or ointment come into contact with the person's eye.
- Ask patient to close eye lightly for a few seconds.
- Wipe away any excess medication that runs down the person's cheek with a clean tissue (one tissue to be used for one wipe only from nose to ear).
- Replace cap (avoid touching the top of the medicine container).
- Wash and dry hands.

Administering ear drops

- Arrange clean tissues or swabs to hand.
- Follow normal patient/medication checks.
- Wash and dry hands.
- Remove cap from container; do not touch the opened top.
- Gently pull the pinna of the ear upwards and backwards taking care not to touch the skin with the dropper.

- Apply drops, taking care not to come in direct contact with the skin.
- Release the pinna.
- Wipe away excess medication with the tissue.
- Wash and dry hands.

HINTS

See Nursing and Midwifery Council's *Standards for Medicines Management* published August 2007 www.nmc-uk.org

Food safety

- Food poisoning is caused by eating contaminated food; this food has been infected with pathogens.
- Food can become contaminated anywhere in the food handling chain. This includes; production, preparation, storage, cooking and eating.
- Bacteria that cause food poisoning include *salmonella, campylobacter* and *e. coli.* The food can be infected directly (by bacteria already present in the food) or indirectly (from contamination from things such as dirty hands or equipment).
- One in ten people in the UK will have food poisoning each year.
- Certain groups of people are more vulnerable to the effects of food poisoning; these groups include older people:
  - babies and young children;
  - pregnant women and unborn babies;
  - people who have multiple health conditions or who are already unwell or who have a suppressed immunity.

■ FOOD REGULATIONS

There are a number of regulations and laws to protect the public from food poisoning. These include:

Protecting the public
- Food Safety Act 1990
- Food Safety (General Food Hygiene) Regulation 1995
- Food Hygiene Regulations (2006)
- Food Standards Agency set up in 2000; this is an independent group responsible for protecting and advising the public

---

■ HANDLING FOOD

Points to consider when handling food:

Hygiene and food:
- equipment;
- personal hygiene;
- food hygiene;
- environment.

Food handling:
- universal precautions.

Food storage:
- temperature;
- use by dates;
- raw foods being stored separately from cooked foods;
- avoiding spillages and contamination.

Food preparation:
- thawing – follow instructions;
- cooking – follow instructions;

- reheating – once only;
- use by dates;
- rinsing vegetables and fruit in cold running water.

Reference / Adapted from Tribal Education (2006) *NCFE Certificate in Infection Control*, York: Tribal.

Urinary catheter management

■ INSERTION OF CATHETERS

- Gain consent.
- Ensure privacy and dignity throughout procedure.
- Use sterile catheterisation pack.
- Use aseptic technique when inserting catheters.
- Inflate catheter balloon using sterile water (use sterile syringe to insert water).
- Clean technique can be adopted for intermittent self catheterisation.

■ CATHETER CARE

- Clean vulval area from above downward using warm soapy water (female patients).
- Retract foreskin before cleaning for male patients so shaft of catheter can be cleaned (replace foreskin following cleaning).
- Rinse well and dry area with a towel.
- Do not allow catheter bag to drag onto the floor: attach to the person, bed or chair using appropriate means.

■ EMPTYING A CATHETER BAG

- Use a jug set aside for this.
- Wash and dry hands.
- Wear gloves and apron.
- Hold bag over edge of bed, open drainage port – make sure drainage port does not touch the jug or the floor or your hands.
- Close drainage port, attach catheter bag as appropriate.
- Dispose of urine in sluice/toilet.
- Clean or discard the urine jug according to local policy.

Reference / Adapted from Nicol, M., Bavin, C. and Bedford-Turner, S. (2004) *Essential Nursing Skills*, St. Louis, MO: Mosby.

The NICE guidelines for the Prevention of Infection (2003) recommend that the following is incorporated into local policies and guidelines for the management of urinary catheters.

Managing urinary catheters
- education of patients, carers and healthcare workers in all relevant aspects of the management of catheter drainage;
- assessment of the need for the use of catheters;
- selecting the type of drainage;
- insertion of the catheter;
- catheter care and maintenance.

Reference / National Institute for Health and Clinical Excellence (2003) *Guidelines for Infection Control*, London: NICE.

■ EDUCATING PATIENTS, CARERS AND HEALTHCARE WORKERS

- The above should all be trained in effective hand washing and decontamination, how to insert intermittent catheters (if applicable) and how to manage catheters. If possible this should take place before the patient is discharged from hospital.
- Any community and primary health and social care staff involved with the person's care should be trained in catheter insertion (if applicable), including suprapubic catheterisation, and in catheter management.
- Follow up training and support for long term catheter management must be in place.

■ ASSESSING THE NEED FOR CATHETERS

- Alternative treatment options should be explored.
- The need for a catheter should be reviewed regularly.
- Any changes to the catheter care and management should be documented.

■ THINGS TO CONSIDER WHEN SELECTING DRAINAGE OPTIONS

- the clinical need (this should be assessed and reviewed regularly);
- the anticipated duration of the need for a catheter (this can affect the type of drainage option selected);
- the person's preference (some people prefer the use of intermittent catheters to indwelling ones);
- assessing the risk of infection and finding ways to minimise this;

- the use of intermittent catheterisation in preference to indwelling;
- the type and size of catheters used (this is determined by each individual person's needs);
- the catheter balloon to be inflated with 10 ml of sterile water for adults and 3–5 ml of sterile water for children;
- valve system to be used in preference to drainage bag;
- indwelling catheters to be inserted using aseptic technique by trained practitioners who have been assessed to do this;
- clean procedure used for intermittent catheter use, single patient lubricant to be used for non-lubricated catheters;
- the meatus to be cleaned before insertion of catheter, in accordance with local policy;
- appropriate lubricant to be used from a single-use container in order to minimise trauma and infection.

■ CATHETER MANAGEMENT

- Connect indwelling catheters to a sterile closed urinary drainage system (a bag) or valve.
- Healthcare staff should ensure that the connection between the catheter and the bag or valve should not be broken except for clinical need. Change bags in accordance with manufacturer's instructions.
- Apply appropriate hand hygiene at all times. Health and social care workers should wash hands and wear single use non-sterile gloves when they are caring for the catheter. Disgard gloves after use and hands washed/ decontaminated.
- The person and their carers should be instructed in the above.

- Obtain urine samples through the sampling port using an aseptic technique.
- Bags should be below the bladder, but not in contact with the floor.
- A link system should be in place to facilitate overnight drainage – this will keep the original system intact.
- Empty the bag frequently to maintain flow and the valve should be released regularly. This prevents reflux and minimises the risk of infection and damage to the kidneys.
- Wash the meatus daily using soap and water.
- Each person should have an individual plan of care and treatment so blockage and encrustation can be minimised. Any tendency to these should be documented.
- Bladder washouts should not be used to prevent catheter associated infections.
- Change catheters when clinically indicated or in accordance with the manufacturer's instructions.
- Give antibiotics prophylactically if a person has a history of catheter associated infections or if they have a heart condition such as heart valve insertion, septal defect, patent ductus or a prosthetic valve.
- Clean reusable, intermittent catheters with soap and water and store dry in accordance with the manufacturer's instructions.

Reference / National Institute for Health and Clinical Excellence (2003) *Guidelines for Infection Control*, London: NICE.

Enteral feeding

Enteral feeding includes naso-gastric feeds and feeding via a percutaneous endoscopic gastrostomy (PEG) tube. Follow standard principles for controlling infection; maintaining scrupulous hand hygiene, wearing personal protective equipment such as aprons and gloves and the correct disposal of waste (including sharps).

■ EDUCATION OF PATIENTS, CARERS AND HEALTH AND SOCIAL CARE WORKERS

This must take place before the person leaves hospital; all those involved need to feel confident and supported. Any further training or updates should take place when required. The person and their carers need to be supported throughout and they need to know where to go for information and advice should they require it.

■ PREPARATION AND STORAGE OF FEEDS

Manufacturer's recommendations should be followed. Whenever possible pre-packaged ready to use feeds should be used. If other types of feeds are used (i.e. those that need reconstituting or diluting) the manufacturer's recommendations must be followed plus the following:
- minimal handling;
- hand hygiene maintained;
- environment in which the feeds are reconstituted or diluted should be clean;

- cooled boiled water or sterile water should be used to dilute or reconstitute;
- no touch technique should be used.

All feeds need to be stored as recommended by the manufacturer:
- the right temperature;
- feeds prepared in advance should be stored in the fridge and in accordance with the manufacturer's instructions. They should be used within 24 hours.

■ ADMINISTRATION OF FEEDS

- minimal handling;
- no touch technique;
- follow manufacturer's recommendations and your organisation's policies and procedures;
- seek advice from dietician, infection control team and manufacturer if necessary.

■ INSERTION SITE

- Wash the stoma daily with soap and water and dry thoroughly.
- Tube should be flushed through with fresh tap water before and after feeding and before and after administering medication to prevent blockage.
- If person has a low immunity – cooled freshly boiled water or sterile water from a freshly opened container should be used.

Reference / National Institute for Health and Clinical Excellence (2003) *Guidelines for Infection Control*, London: NICE.

■ DECONTAMINATING ENTERAL FEEDING PUMP

- Consult and follow local policy and guidelines.
- Wipe with detergent and warm water.
- Dry.
- Wipe with 70% alcohol if contaminated with blood.

HINT
This applies to most electrical equipment. Take care when wiping down electrical equipment.

Central venous catheters

Central venous catheters are used to administer fluids, medicines, blood components and for total parenteral nutrition. The standard principles should be followed (see above). For haemodialysis patients follow the recommendations of the dialysis centres.

■ POINTS TO CONSIDER

- education of patients, carers and health and social care workers;
- general asepsis;
- catheter site care;
- standard principles for catheter management.

Your responsibilities as an employee

As an employee in a healthcare setting you have a responsibility to minimise the risks of infection and to manage any infection.

Your responsibilities as an employee
- Take professional and personal responsibility for your own working practices.
- Protect yourself and others from the risks of infection.
- Use standard universal precautions.
- Follow your organisation's policies and procedures for infection control.
- Ensure you are up to date with developments in this subject.
- Attend relevant training.
- Ensure you are fit to work.

Your employer's responsibilities

Your employer has a responsibility to ensure that their employees are safe from the risks of infection and any infection is managed appropriately.

The employer's responsibility for infection control
- Make sure all employees understand any infection risks and know how to take appropriate action.
- Ensure all legal regulations are followed (such as the Health and Safety at Work Act.
- Protect employees and others from risks of infection.
- Ensure policies and procedures are up to date and relevant.